Carb Cycling For Athletes: How To Cycle Carbohydrates for Maximum Performance

Mark Brave

Contents

Introduction

Before I get into who I am I just wanted to take a minute to explain why I decided to write this book. There are a lot of nutrition books out there, that all have there place and can be great, but none of these books are actually written by a strength athlete who competes in performance sports. I also feel like a lot of these books don't include a detailed plan for what you should do on a year long plan. I've been strength training and competing in strongman, crossfit, adventure races, and now powerlifting. Throughout the years I've studied nutrition throughout college, through books, and from working with some of the best nutritionist in the game. I know nutrition is a huge component to improving body composition and to dramatically improve sports performance that is always so confusing for the average person.

Through my years of working with people and myself I've come up with a simplified way to make this complicated diet stuff work for you. I continue to learn and educate myself so that I can always be up to date with the latest science, but I will always refer back to what I have done and whats been done before me with great results. I take science with anecdotal bro science and mix it together in a complete comprehensive book for you to learn and grow. I recommend you do the same, be your own science experiment and try new things and actually give it a chance to work

I will also like to say that not any one diet will fit all body types. It ultimately comes down to trial and error and figuring out what approach/plan works best for you and the one you can see yourself doing for a long time. Because at the end of the day the plan you can stick to the longest will yield the greatest results.

CHAPTER 1: NUTRITION 101

The body thrives when properly fueled, think of it as a high powered sports car you put the best oiil and gas in it so it runs smoothly. You keep the brakes and transmission running smooth and constantly checked. You have the best tires on it so it can handle the sharp turns and crazy amount of horsepower. Now imagine if one of those things gets out of whack or neglected the car slowly starts to break down and under perform just like the human body when you feed it trash and not the fuel it needs. How you treat your body plays a huge role in how it performs, so forget about those days of McDonalds and twinkies. Proper training programs, sleep, stress, and nutrition, they all play a huge role in how your body performs but one is not more important than the other they all have to work synergistically in order for you to perform at an optimal level. The best way to know why it works so well is to learn what happens when you eat macros and what each macro brings to the table. So here is your nutrition 101 down to the basics.

.

The Basics

Your body needs energy to perform the tasks we ask of it. Calories equals energy for the body and calories are made up of proteins, carbs, and fats. Over the years I am sure you've heard bad things about all 3 of these and hence the advent of so many gimmicky diets that takes one out and says its the worst thing for you and you are not reaching your goals because of it... Seriously the best snake oil propaganda ever, the scare tactic to make you buy their diet is just getting ridiculous. I am here to tell you that you need them all and here is why:

Carbs give you energy and replenishes your used glycogen stores which help transport a lot of your protein and other micronutrients such as vitamins and minerals to keep your body functioning at a high level. Carbs will help with the restoration of glycogen stores that have been depleted due to intense workouts. Carbs are also the most metabolic nutrient we eat. The are a key macro nutrient for a diet as it is protein sparing so it will help preserve size and give you energy around your workouts. For every gram of carbohydrates you consume it equates to 4 calories.

Fats are great at regulating hormones such as testosterone, thyroid, and others, they also help suppress hunger as you diet which is crucial to staying on track. Fats are also good at keeping you fuller longer, reduces cortisol levels, provides energy, and assist in the body functioning properly. It also helps with insulin sensitivity and cardiovascular health. Fats are extremely important while dieting, naturally as you go   into a calorie deficit your testosterone and other hormones down regulate so the fats will keep your endocrine system healthier. It also helps with joint pain which will come as you get leaner. For every gram of fat you consume it equates to 9 calories.

Proteins are the building block of muscle growth and repair so after a hard workout protein breaks down into amino acids and begin the repair process so you can make it back the next day and kill your next workout. Protein also has the highest thermogenic effect on the body meaning it burns the most calories of all the macros   when you consume it.

Protein is also great at keeping you satiated/full longer. So as you can see protein is crucial for successful dieting it not only helps you keep on your muscle, but it also plays a huge role in burning calories and keeping you full all things that will help any dieter stay sane. For every gram of protein you consume it equates to 4 calories.

So as you can see they all play an important role in your fitness journey and neglecting anyone completely is just a bad idea and isn't necessary so why do it?

Chapter 2: A diet that works

As stated earlier the diet you can stick to the longest is the one that will yield the best results, but a diet without knowledge is not a very wise choice. I've had several clients contacting me wondering why they can't lose weight and I ask to see their diet and all the food on there is healthy and their compliance is high so what gives? Its a lot about placing and timing of macronutrients that will make a diet as effective as it should be.

First and foremost you have to figure out the amount calories you need to consume. You can do this several ways but in all reality it comes down to trial and error. I recommend just taking your bodyweight and multiplying it by 10x if you are sedentary, by 12x if you're active, and by 15x if you have a manual labor job and are active. This will be a good baseline for you, now everybody is different so it may take some tinkering to figure out what calorie point works for you but give this a try for a week and see what happens.

Once you have the calories down, let's move onto the macros. Before we do I want to simplify things as much as possible so if I say protein for 21g which is around 3oz of meat, 20g of carbs which is 1/2 cup of cooked brown rice, and 8g of fat which is around 1tblsp of almond butter. Now if your fat has protein and carbs thats fine don't count it and this goes for all the other macros as well. A protein is just a protein, fats are fats, etc... Now with that being said if it is a low fat meal try to keep it leaner meats such as cod, skinless chicken breast, etc.. If its a fat meal you can add red meat or fattier meat, but be aware of it and if the scale isn't moving it may be because you are eating to much fattier meat.

Next on the list of importance is protein per day you should be eating per day this does not change for training days and non training days. I like to go a bit higher then recommended so for males go bet 1.2-1.5g per pound of bodyweight and for females go with .8-1.2g per pound of bodyweight. The reason behind the discrepancy is that no matter what females just don't carry as much muscle and tend to carry more body fat.

They will not need to push the protein envelope any higher simply because their bodies can't readily use it as much as the males body can.

So now that you have that figured out, next you need to find an adequate amount of meals you can eat per day. Now I know it comes down to a lot of times calories in versus calories out but what the research shows and what has been proven to be extremely effective for keeping muscle on and hunger levels normal during a diet is   more meals per day. So 5-6 meals per day is the ideal marker, some may need 7-8 others can go as low as 4 but I highly recommend at least 5. The reason behind the smaller more frequent meals is "Nutrient timing incorporates the use of methodical planning and eating of whole foods, nutrients extracted from food, and other sources.

The timing of the energy intake and the ratio of certain ingested macronutrients are likely the attributes which allow for enhanced recovery and tissue repair following high- volume exercise, augmented muscle protein synthesis, and improved mood states when compared with unplanned or traditional strategies of nutrient intake." John Meadows

So now let's break down protein into an evenly divided number for meals. An example is a 200lbs male eating 240g of protein per day will have a meal breakdown that looks like this:

Meal 1

40g of Protein

Meal 2

40g of Protein

Meal 3

40g of Protein

Meal 4

40g of Protein

Meal 5

40g of Protein

Meal 6

40g of Protein

So 240g of protein gives us 960 calories. For an active 200lbs male who's baseline of calories is 2400, this leaves us with 1440 calories for the rest of our macros. So this is roughly 40% of our daily calorie breakdown.

Onto carbohydrates next, now these along with fats will vary on training and non training days and I will get into the how's and why's behind that a little later. Right now we are just trying to find our baseline. For baseline I like to go with 35% carbohydrates, so that gives us 210g of carbs for the day at 840 calories. So a simplified breakdown of that without looking into training, non training, and timing would look like this.

Meal 1

40g of Protein

35g of Carbohydrates

Meal 2

40g of Protein

35g of Carbohydrates

Meal 3

40g of Protein

35g of Carbohydrates

Meal 4

40g of Protein

35g of Carbohydrates

Meal 5

40g of Protein

35g of Carbohydrates

Meal 6

40g of Protein

35g of Carbohydrates

Last but not least are the fats and these just make up the rest of your total calorie intake which is at 600 calories once we add up the carbs and proteins. So the fat for the day is 67g of fat at 600 calories. This is a pretty simple way to get things started and in all honesty you can run this and still see results without worrying about a thing like nutrient timing, training day nutrition, etc.. but it wouldn't be the most optimal way and if you're reading this book you are looking to become the best. So here is the final meal breakdown.

Meal 1

40g of Protein

35g of Carbohydrates

11g of Fat

Meal 2

40g of Protein

35g of Carbohydrates

11g of Fat

Meal 3

40g of Protein

35g of Carbohydrates

11g of Fat

Meal 4

40g of Protein

35g of Carbohydrates

11g of Fat

Meal 5

40g of Protein

35g of Carbohydrates

11g of Fat

Meal 6

40g of Protein

35g of Carbohydrates

11g of Fat

Pretty simple, right? I could just end the book there collect my money and send you on your merry way, but there is so much more to it, to become the best you can be. Sure any plan will work and if you're just trying to lose a few pounds you don't really have to read any further you know why macros are important and what the body uses them for and you know how to write and calculate a good base plan. Basically that's all you need to shed off a few pounds or to try and gain a few. Now if your goal is to achieve things that are seem out of reach or if you're trying to maximize your potential than the rest of these chapters are what really matters.

Chapter 3: Nutrient timing: when, how often, and what to eat

Nutrient timing has been around forever, but it wasn't until recently that its gained a ton of popularity. The timing of nutrients is crucial for any athlete looking to drop a weight class or to simply perform at an optimal level. Nutrient timing is about when to eat, how often to eat, and what to eat. I will discuss the ins and outs of this concept in the simplest form so that all you'll have to do is read it once and you'll never forget it, well maybe.

How often you should eat really plays a large role in energy, mood, and body composition. Breaking your calories down into several small meals a day has the benefit of consistent blood spikes so your energy is controlled, less hunger throughout the day which will prevent you from splurging or overeating, and it's been show through years of bodybuilding and now backed by some science that it will change your body   composition to a more favorable leaner you.

Now several meals throughout the day works for most and quite honestly should work for everyone, but you will always have that job or life get in the way. Are these excuses? Quite frankly yes, if you want something bad enough you'll make it happen. Nonetheless this will come up so I'll throw in some pointers and tips to help you reach your goals just in case you can't eat 5-6 meals per day.

- Tip Number 1: If you can only eat 3-4x a day supplement with a shake or a BCAA's drink in bet meals.
- Tip Number 2: If there is an extended period bet meals and you're hungry either drink coffee or chew gum, this will help with appetite.
- Tip Number 3: Eat plenty of

veggies with meals as this will slow down digesting and increase satiety.
- Tip Number 4: Have a healthy snack drawer at work with things like tuna, beef jerky, or other sources of protein.
- Tip Number 5: When in doubt eat protein and veggies, snacking on veggies in between meals is also a viable option.

Basically from the time you wake until the time you sleep you should eat every 2 1/2-3 1/2 hours. Whether it be in the form of a whole meal or shake it doesn't matter something is better than nothing. Timing would be complete if I didn't mention the timing of your peri workout drink, peri workout meaning pre, during, and after, this drink should start to be consumed 20-30 minutes before the workout just sipping it and then drink all of it throughout your workout. After the shake is done your post workout meal can be consumed 45-90 minutes afterwards.

Now that we have our meals and timing planned out let's talk about the timing of macronutrients such as carbs, fats, and proteins.

No matter what diet you do these priceless reign true, so if you are carb cycling, zone, paleo, or flexible dieting these concepts will help you establish the criteria for putting your meals together.

Let's start with protein first. Protein is the building blocks of muscles and must be eaten at every meal, but some proteins are bester than others and some are just more appropriate for the timing of the meal. First lets start with during and after the workout, you want a fast absorbing a digesting protein during the workout so a whey isolate is preferred, anyone just find the brand that has the lowest fat and carbs in it and that sits well with your stomach. Post workout go with a mix of casein and whey this will provide you with a fast and slower digesting protein which will help you sustain protein synthesis longer which is the repair and building of muscles. As far as a post workout meal goes if you are dropping carbs than red meat is preferred as it has a better amino acid profile than white meat but if carbs stay high then go with a less fatty meat such as any white meat. Thats pretty much the standard for all meals outside of this window. If carbs are high go with more white or leaner meats and if carbs are low or you're not adding in any fats than go with a red meat. For bedtime you want a slower digesting protein, so something like casein or dairy works great here just be residents of the calories you   don't want to go to bed with a full belly as it may mess with your sleep.

Next up is the dreaded carbs, they have such a bad rap but can do so many great things for performance and body composition. Instead of using things like the Glycemic Index to describe carbs we will just go with fast digesting carbs and slow digesting carbs.

The more processed the faster the carbs digest, think things like cereal, cream of rice, baby food etc.. these simple carbs are great to eat before and after a workout and when I say before and after I mean 20-30 minutes before and after. It's not uncommon for me to eat 3-4 rice krispie treats and a shake before hitting the gym. The reason behind this is 1. you don't want a bunch of food sitting in your stomach while your training and 2. the faster you digest it the faster it starts to circulate through your bloodstream to promote muscle building and recovery.

Slow digesting carbs are great to eat at any other meal throughout the day,   things like brown rice, oatmeal, sweet potatoes, etc… are slower digesting so the insulin spike is not as high and it will give your longer more sustainable energy throughout the day. They are also great at keeping you fuller longer so when on a cut these are great to add so you're not starving meal to meal.

Next question is when should I eat my carbs and that really depends on your   goal and when exactly you train. The 3 times of the day when carbs will elicit the   greatest response is the 1st meal of the day, pre workout, and post workout. This is when you insulin receptors are the most sensitive to the absorption of carbs. If your insulin isn't sensitive and more resistant then a lot of your carbs will help shuttle nutrients to your fat cells as opposed to your muscle glycogen stores. Now if your goal is to gain weight carbs are great to have at every meal just the quantity gets ramped up around the workout and lowered at other times away from your workout. Here as a breakdown of the same meal plan above but with the separation for timing:

Meal 1

40g of Protein

40g of Carbohydrates

5 g of fat

Meal 2

40g of Protein

20g of Carbohydrates

16 g of fat

Meal 3

40g of Protein

20g of Carbohydrates

16 g of fat

Meal 4 Pre Workout

40g of Protein

50g of Carbohydrates

2 g of fat

Meal 5 Post Workout

40g of Protein

65g of Carbohydrates

2 g of fat

Meal 6

40g of Protein

15g of Carbohydrates

23 g of fat

So as you can see the last thing covered is fats and I keep fats lower when carbs are higher. This is due to when carbs are consumed they spike your insulin and when fats are eaten with carbs you have more of a chance to get nutrients shuttled to fat cells more so than to muscle cells. I also keep fats the lowest around the workout window, fats also slow down digesting which is not what we want going on around the workout we want our nutrients absorbed fast and to be ready to use immediately.

Now that you know how to organize things and the reasons behind it, it will only take a few minor adjustments to get them dialed in. Without a shadow of a doubt food is the most important thing so before you move onto supplements make sure you're set on food first or else you're just wasting your time and money.

This brings me to my last point on nutrient timing, veggies are great and should definitely be consumed and as long as they are fibrous they are not counted as part of your macros. Fibrous meaning the carb to fiber ratio is close to identical. They are great at filling space in your stomach when dieting and they have a lot of great vitamin/mineral benefits as well. With that being said I also keep them away from pre and post workout meals for the simple fact that they slow things down.

CHAPTER 4: DO SUPPLEMENTS REALLY WORK?

Supplements the magic elixir that's going to put you over the top, turn you into the best right?? Probably not, if you're relying on supplements to do the work you will probably never make it to the top, but nevertheless there are a few supplements that have stood the test of time and can be extremely effective in helping you in your performance and physique goals. Like I said before food first but here is a list of a few supplements that I really like:

- Creatine
- Protein Powder
- BCAA's
- L Leucine
- L Glutamine

- Highly Branched Cyclic Dextrins
- Fish Oil
- Borage Oil
- R-ALA

Creatine is a supplement that has been around for decades and has always been scientifically proven to work at increasing strength and lean body mass. Your body relies on creatine to produce action of the muscles when lifting weights so supplementing your pre or intra workout supplement with 5-10g of creatine will help with recovery time and allow you to squeeze out a few more reps. You can also get creatine from steak and all other red meats. This is a good supplement that will help you perform better in the gym. I get a very basic creatine monohydrate and at 240lbs take 10g during training and 5g on non training days. Also is you add 1/3tsp of baking soda with the creatine it will magnify the results of creatine even more. I prefer any brand that is just a micronized creatine monohydrate, I get mine from Dymatize.

Protein powder comes in all shapes and sizes. A lot of new research has come out stating how bad some of the popular brands of protein actually are. A lot of companies use bcaa fillers to equate to their protein labels which makes the actual protein bioavailability small. So finding the right kind is extremely important and this is also why   I prefer whole food over protein powders. Some good reputable brands are Optimum, Nature's Best, TrueNutrition, Dymatize, and SlingShot. I recommend two different types of proteins, whey isolate and casein.

Whey Isolates is a fast absorbing protein which is great to drink pre, during, and post workout. It hits your blood stream fast and is typically easy to digest so it won't cause any gut irritation. When looking for a good whey look for something that is low in fat and carbs. A few brands that I recommend are Dymatize Iso 100, Natures Best Isopure, Slingshot Protein, and Animal Whey.

Casein is a slower digesting protein and is great to use throughout the day but best to use right before bed. The delayed release will allow your body to use the nutrients throughout the night while you sleep. So they will help spare a lot of muscle breakdown from being in a fasted state while sleeping. A few brands I like are Universal Casein, Dymatize Elite Casein, Ultimate Nutrition Casein.

BCAA's are a great supplement to add to your pre, during, and post workout shakes. Plus if you're cutting weight and are hungry in between meals a BCAA drink will not only suppress appetite but it will allow you to preserve more muscle while dieting. When you eat protein it is broken down into amino acids to be used/synthesized by your muscles for repair and growth. BCAA's are just a free form of amino acids that can supplement your protein intake and help with the rebuilding process after a brutal workout. Taking bet 5-10g peri workout is a good start. Amino Energy On, Prime Nutrition BCAA's are two great brands.

L Leucine as a standalone amino acid has been shown to have more of an increase to protein synthesis than any of the other ones. Meaning that its more anabolic in nature. Leucine also activates mTOR which manufactures muscle proteins to help in the building process. This is a must supplement while dieting as it has been shown to help you lose weight while maintaining muscle mass. Serving size can be anywhere from

3-10g depending on when you take it and with what you take with it. All Max Nutrition, Prime Nutrition, Dymatize are great brands.

L Glutamine provides 1/3 of the bodies nitrogen which will help with nitrogen balance throughout the body. Which helps you recover from muscle damage from workouts. It helps improve with digestion as well along with the absorption of food. Take around

10-15g per day and bump it up when in high stress periods. Prima force and Dymatize I highly recommend.

Highly Branched Cyclic Dextrins or HBCD are a form of simple carbohydrates that is ideal to consume for your periworkout nutrition. This is a fast digesting carb but what separates them from all the other fast digest carbs on the market is not only does it digest and absorb fast but due to the cone shape molecule it is it has a higher uptake of nutrients and once it settles down into your stomach it holds the nutrients longer   allowing for a longer absorption rate.

So it moves through the body just as fast but it allows your nutrients to get fully distributed before we get rid of them through waste.

The great thing about spiking your insulin during and after a workout is two fold. One it helps the blunt the process of muscle breakdown, so its easier to recover from workout to workout. Second it helps speed up the process of muscle repair by shuttling nutrients through your body to induce protein synthesis at a faster rate. Buy these at Truenutrition.com, discount code geared

Fish Oil is a great tool to fight off inflammation caused by hard workouts, this will allow for better recovery. It has also been show to help promote protein synthesis. It increases insulin sensitivity and cardiac output and stroke volume which promotes a healthy heart. Now Ultimate Omegas, Nordics, Jarrow are 3 terrific brands.

Borage Oil is a great fat for the same reasons as fish oil above but it is a fat that actual helps you burn fat. It also has anti inflammatory properties to it. It may help with eczema, asthma, and arthritis. Now Borage is great.

LA is a glucose disposal aid, that helps shuttle nutrients, specifically carbs to the muscle instead of fat stores. This is a great supplement to take if you are having a high carb meal. It also is a powerful indirect anti oxidation method that rapidly regenerates other endogenous antioxidants. All Max Nutrition is a great brand.

So now that we went over the supplements that I recommend and I only recommend them after you have all your food, sleep, and training down. Let's put them together to form our peri workout nutrition, this is a supplement drink that I use to help keep muscle from breaking down, building muscle faster and giving you energy throughout your workout. Peri workout is pre, during, and after supplement nutrition that you start to drink 20-30minutes pre workout, drinking 2/3 during the workout and the rest after the workout is done.

For the shake I use a big jug of water and fill it half way up and just pour everything in there. As stated above I like a 4:1 ration of carbs to protein for this shake so for our 200lbs athlete who requires 30g of protein will need 120g of carbs. So the shake will look like this:

- 30g of protein
- 10g of BCAA's
- 10g of Creatine
- 5g of L Leucine
- 120g of HBCD

This is something you will tinker with a few times to get it down but this guideline should help you get started.

CHAPTER 5: MATCHING NUTRITION TO YOUR TRAINING

Your diet should match the amount of work done per day. It drives me nuts to see people eat the same food day in and day out without taking into consideration the amount of work done for the day. When setting up your diet I like to do a carb cycling approach that allows you to 1. speed up your metabolism by rotating calories higher to lower and carbs higher to lower. 2. Allows you to have a day to build and a day to burn. Training days you're trying to build muscle and recover so having high carbs on this day will allow for that. Non training days are to burn fat so I lower the carbs up the fat and add in some cardio.

The major reason behind carb cycling being a great approach is it tricks your body while dieting to allow it to shed more fat and weight. As you start a diet your body immediately fights against you to keep homeostasis, because the thought of our body losing fat is the same signaling patterns as if we are starving to death so our body will do everything it can to not starve and die. This is why it is so hard to lose weight sometimes.

The benefits of carb cycling is it tricks the body to allow it to start burning fat again. A high carb day is a great day to build muscle so putting your high carb day on a lagging body part or a max effort day is ideal. How to trick your body to keep burning fat while dieting is to make sure when you have a high carb day to make sure its above maintenance. If you eat below calories on this day than it won't have the same response to your body and the weight will still stale. I recommend starting with 2 high carb days a week with 72hrs separating each one. Your other training days will be medium carb days and on your off days or cardio days will be your low carb days. So an example of how I would set up a few different training templates:

Sunday: Off day, Low Carbs

Monday: Max Effort Upper Body, High Carb Day

Tuesday: Dynamic Effort Lower Body, Medium Carb Day

Wednesday: Off day, Low Carbs

Thursday: Dynamic Effort Upper Body, Medium Carb Day
Friday: Max Effort Lower Body, High Carb Day

Saturday: Off day, Low Carb Day

Sunday: Front Squats and Back, Medium Carb Day

Monday: Pause Bench Day, Medium Carb Day
Tuesday: Squat Day, High Carb Day

Wednesday: Off day, Low Carbs

Thursday: Pause Bench Day, Medium Carb Day

Friday: Deadlift Day, High Carb Day

Saturday: Off day, Low Carb Day

Sunday: Legs, High Carb Day

Monday: Off day, Low Carb Day

Tuesday: Shoulders, Medium Carb Day

Wednesday: Back, Medium Carb Day

Thursday: Off day, Low Carb Day

Friday: Chest, High Carb Day

Saturday: Arms, Medium Carb Day

CHAPTER 6: BUILDING THE MASTER PLAN

Onto the application of everything we've gone over, I am sure most of you just skipped to this, once you look at this please go back and read everything so it makes sense. Now there are so many ways to diet and to do it effectively and I outlined a lot of basic ideas that can help you build a plan based on your personal beliefs and what diet you think will work best for you. I personally prefer to do a carb cycling approach that matches your carbs to the days of training and non training. I will continue to use the same examples as I've done in the previous chapters.

High Carb Day 2640 calories active 200lbs male
Remember this is your day to build muscle and push calories. This day we take our base

calories and multiply it by 10% for our surplus.

Meal 1
42g of Protein
65g of Carbohydrates

Meal 2
42g of Protein
50g of Carbohydrates

Meal 3
42g of Protein
50g of Carbohydrates

Meal 4
42g of Protein
65g of Carbohydrates

Meal 5 Peri Workout 30g of protein
10g of BCAA's 10g of Creatine 5g of L Leucine
120g of HBCD

Meal 6
42g of Protein
70g of Carbohydrates

Medium Carb Day 2160 Calories
This is still a workout day, but the calories will drop 10%, which with the timing of our nutrients we can still be in a calorie deficit to

help lose fat and build muscle because we put out carbs around the workout.

Meal 1
42g of Protein
30g of Carbohydrates 6g of Fat

Meal 2
42g of Protein 15g of Fat

Meal 3
42g of Protein 15g of Fat

Meal 4
42g of Protein
30g of Carbohydrates 6g of Fat

Meal 5 Peri Workout 30g of protein
10g of BCAA's 10g of Creatine 5g of L Leucine 120g of HBCD

Meal 6
42g of Protein
40g of Carbohydrates 3g of Fat

Low Carb Day 1920 Calories

This is our day to burn fat and lose some weight, i prefer doing cardio, recovery workouts, and mobility stuff on this day. This day we drop calories by 20% of our maintenance level.
Meal 1

40g of Protein
20g of Carbohydrates 7g of Fat

Meal 2
40g of Protein
20g of Carbohydrates 7g of Fat

Meal 3
40g of Protein
20g of Carbohydrates 7g of Fat

Meal 4
40g of Protein
0g of Carbohydrates 18g of Fat

Meal 5
40g of Protein
0g of Carbohydrates 18g of Fat

Meal 6
40g of Protein
0g of Carbohydrates 18g of Fat

Once you have your calories set and your macros, you evenly space out your protein through the 6 meals. Place the bulk of your carbs around your workout and everything else is a person to person trial base to find the perfect spot for the rest of your macros. So plug them in based on what I stated earlier and do it for a week and re check weight if you dropped and that's the goal great leave it alone, if you gained or remained the same rearrange them first before you start dropping out some macros.

There will come a time where changes will need to be made, when your weight starts to plateau I would first add HIIT cardio or an extra workout day to see if that drops the weight first. I always prefer to do more to see results before I drop calories because once you drop them there is no turning back. HIIT cardio or high intensity interval training is the preferred method of cardio, it will burn more calories throughout the day with less time involved. Plus it will also help build up muscle and boost recovery with things like sled sprints, stair sprints, or prowler sprints. HIIT cardio is done at an all out pace for a desired time or distance, than full recovery rest before you go again. Start off with 4-5 sprints and then either add more sprints each week or reduce rest time to make progress.

Now if you added more work in and things have hit a wall again than its a simple process of removing macros. First macro to remove will be your fats, take off 5% for each day for a week. If the scale drops awesome leave things alone until you plateau again. If you hit a wall again, next drop 5% carbs, Now with fats you can remove them from your carb meals first before taken them out of your low to no carb meals and with carbs you take them out of the meals furthest away from you workout. You just keep rotating this process until you reach your desired goals. Its literally that simple.

Another approach as you get longer into the diet is to start dropping days, So instead of having 2 high carb days you can drop to 1, and replace it with a medium day. Same thing for medium days just drop 1 day to a low carb day.

There will come a point in time where you've been dieting and things are going great and then all of a sudden you hit a wall and you can't seem to pass through it. Here is a little tip to get you through that plateau.

Dieting is a hard endeavor and it is extremely frustrating at times. You want to see the scale move down and you want it to move down fast. When you are doing everything right and it still doesn't go down you start to second guess why the hell am I doing this. So you lower the calories a little more and you add in some more cardio and a week later still nothing. What is going on here?

Once you start a diet and you begin a calorie deficit, because lets face it the 2 ways to lose weight is to consume less or exercise more, your body starts to immediately work against to maintain status quo or homeostasis. Your body likes it were it is and doesn't want to help you in your goal to lose weight. Once the diet starts your testosterone will drop, your metabolic rate will start to slow and your body will send all kinds of useless signals to you that it is starving and you need to eat more.

After a period of time your body pretty much fights so hard that you start to plateau as stated in the first chapter. So what do you do? Add more cardio? Lift more weights? Lower calories even more? All these can possibly get you back on track or they can create a more stressful environment for your body and stress creates cortisol and with high levels of cortisol floating around it becomes a real pain in the ass to lose weight.

The answer is to eat more!!! And more specifically eat more carbs!! I know you like the sound of that. The refeed day is a one day a a week high carb, extremely low fat day that will help balance your body and to let it know you're not starving and are not going to die and that its ok to let go of some more body fat. This will also help the uptick of leptin, why is that important for people trying to lose weight. Martin Berkhan describes leptin in an article "In the long-term, leptin is regulated by total amount of fat mass. A drop in leptin affects the other hormones negatively and vice versa. Low leptin leads to an increase in hunger and a decrease in metabolic rate, much like high leptin leads to a decrease in hunger and an increase in metabolic rate." So as you're dieting and getting leaner your leptin drops which drops your metabolic rate and makes you hungry. The refeed day is a great way to boost leptin and to allow your body to start dropping fat again.

These refeeds are only for people who have been dieting for an extended period of time and who have become somewhat lean, so don't start this on day one of your diet. The way I like to approach these days is to have half your carbs be from starchy sources and the other half be from extremely low fat sugary sources such as cereal, fat free frozen yogurts, low fat baked goods, pancakes, etc... You also want to make sure that you are in a calorie surplus as well. So lets say you have 100g of carbs on the regular diet, on the reseed days I would bump it to 300g and if you make progress on the scale the next week bump it up a little more. I also recommend doing the refeed on training days as well. Try this out if your diet is plateauing.

45

CHAPTER 7: BULKING OR CUTTING

It seems nowadays everybody wants to be jacked and tan, well I am here to tell you that sometimes you need to just get big, strong, and FLUFFY. If you are always on a quest to get lean and wondering why your lifts aren't going up, but hey you look good with your shirt off right? So than why the hell do you compete in a sport that the strongest person wins, not the leanest or the tannest but the one who can lift the most weight possible. If you're reading this and think who cares about being that strong I   want to look good and be kinda strong so i can get all the likes on instagram then   maybe you should actually compete in a BB or physique show where looks matter. Now I'm not saying go to the store everyday and eat all the chocolate bars and ice cream,   but you will be eating that stuff if you really want to gain some weight. Adding muscle and size is extremely hard to come by if you can add albs of muscle to your frame a year you're lucky, but take any person and you can drop 20-30lbs in a 8-12 week diet. So its time to put up your squeems, stop the salads and cardio and get ready to get huge and strong.

We've all heard it you gotta eat big to get big and that is the truth, you have to eat and consume a massive amount of food in order to grow, sometimes to the point of   force feeding. Now I know this sounds appealing to some of you but its not as fun as it sounds. All you start to think about is food it consumes you. You can go about this in two ways you can eat anything and everything in sight and just get there right away or you can be a little more methodical in your approach and gain at a steady and progressive manner. In this article we will talk about both methods as I definitely feel they both have there benefits and can both yield the results you want over time. Always keep in mind and this is the hardest thing for some lifters is that any approach you take to gaining weight and adding size you will ALWAYS accumulate some fat, so if you're an   endomorph get mentally ready for the struggle of feeling "fat".

The eat everything and anything approach was an extremely popular approach back when geared lifting was king and all anybody cared about was being huge and strong. If you look at the a lot of the top lifters in the sport they eat a lot and they eat almost anything they want, because our sport requires calories aka energy to perform are task where these calories come from is not as important on this approach just that they are there. Clearly these trailblazers make sure protein is the cornerstone of their diet but they also know that eating 5,000-6,000 calories a day of clean food is no small task and can be a daunting one so they supplement with high calorie foods like ice cream, pizza, pasta, and the occasional cheesecake and by occasional I mean everyday!! Now if you have the genetics and/or the right kind of supplements you can stay lean as do some of the top lifters tend to do or if your genetics are lacking you will start to look doughy but that is ok as our sport it's not about how you look but who is the strongest. Let me say that again its not about how you look but who is the strongest. So a day of eating on this approach will be a lot of protein throughout, an occasional junk food, tons of carbs and anything else you can fit down your gullet before you go to bed. This is just a rough ex of 220lbs athlete:

Dirtier Day Meal 1:
4-5 Pancakes with Syrup 4-5 Whole Eggs Sausage and Bacon

Meal 2: Snickers Bar
Big Glass of Milk

Meal 3:
2 Chipotle Burritos Gatorade

Meal 4:
PB&J's
Big Glass of Milk

Meal 5:
Large Meat Lovers Pizza Some Cookies

Bedtime:
Big Bowl of Ice Cream Protein Shake

Cleaner Day Meal 1:
Biscuits
4-5 Whole Eggs Omelet with lots of Meat

Meal 2: Protein Shake 4tbsp of PB
Banana

Meal 3:
Burgers and some Fries Gatorade

Meal 4:
2 Protein Bars Big Glass of Milk

Meal 5:
Chicken Parmesan Gatorade

Bedtime:
2 cups of Chocolate Milk Protein Shake

The pros and cons of this approach are kinda obvious but lets break it down anyways. Pros are you get to eat whatever you want to get the scale moving upwards, you'll gain weight at an exceptional rate, you'll get strong as hell, and you get to wear sweat pants and flip flops year round. The cons are you'll gain a lot of fat, it's not the healthier of the two approaches (but our sport isn't healthy when competing at a high level anyways), you may have a hard time doing anything other than lifting weights, and you damn sure won't look good for bikini season. I would say that this approach can be extremely effective if and only if you know when and have the will power to pull the reigns back and tighten things up. Meaning you can gain but so much weight at a giving period of time which will result in actually muscle gains and your body can only handle so much crap before it starts to fight back and create other issues so by doing something like a 3 month eat everything approach and 3-4 week mini diet in between is a good way to go so that your body is able to keep growing in an effective manner that will elicit the response you want. The bad thing is we are powerlifters for a reason we like to eat, so I've seen a lot of people go to far down the rabbit hole on this path and   eat themselves into an undesirable weight class. I feel like this approach is great for someone who can really only commit to eating clean for a short period of time so the mini diets work extremely well for allowing your body to grow, to allow your body to get desensitized to insulin and to allow your body a period of normalization to help fight off some diseases that come along with eating like crap. Now when I say mini diet I don't mean eat at an extreme calorie deficit and lose a bunch of weight that's not our goal I mean to get the crap out and clean things up while maintaining the weight gain you just accumulated.

Bulk Up 12 Weeks

5,000-8,000 Calories

Mini Diet 4 Weeks

3,800-4,500 Calories

Bulk Up 8 Weeks

5,500-8,500 Calories

Mini Diet 2-3 Weeks

4,000-4,750 Calories

Seems like a lot of food? That's because it is and that's what it takes in either approach is food in abundance. The next approach is for the person who can stick to a fairly regimented thing and that knows the better quality food they consume the better their performance will be so they stick to a clean more bodybuilding approach, don't be mistaken thought this is not the mythical lean gains diet that will have you shredded and bigger at the same time, unfortunately that doesn't exist. Any nutrition plan that puts you in a calorie surplus will make you accumulate fat to some extent the amount varies from person to person depending on training age, actual age, drug usage, and genetics. So if you're an endomorph be prepared to get chunky!!!

I like to approach this in a cyclic manner as well but from a day to day perspective and not a weeks to weeks one like the above mentioned plan. So you have your high carb days, medium carb days, and low carb days.

High days will be used on your highest volume days, medium is on all other training days, and low is on your off days. The tricky part when planning this out is making sure the calorie intake within the week, not the day, is in a surplus that elicits weight gain. So an example of this would look like this for a 220lbs athlete.

High Carb Day:

Meals	Protein	Carbs	Fat		
1	40g	100g	0g		
2	40g	75g	0g		
3	40g	75g	0g		
4	40g	75g	0g		
5 Peri Workout		40g	150g	0g	
6	40g	75g	0g		
7	40g	75g	0g		

Medium Carb Day:

Meals	Protein	Carbs	Fat		
1	50g	60g	10g		
2	50g	40g	12g		
3	50g	40g	12g		
4	50g	40g	12g		
5 Peri Workout		40g	150g	0g	
6	50g	60g	8g		
7	50g	0g	15g		

Low Carb Day:

Meals	Protein	Carbs	Fat
1	50g	40g	15g
2	50g	20g	15g

3	50g	20g	15g
4	50g	20g	15g
5	50g	20g	15g
6	50g	20g	15g
7	50g	0g	20g

This is the approach I prefer for several reasons, one of which is how you eat will most definitely affect how you will perform in the gym. Also how you eat will affect the way you look and your muscles look. So the food quality is equally important as the amount, so yes a calorie is a calorie but if you think 100 calories of Lucky Charms will contribute to performance the same as 100 calories of sweet potato just ask your a high level bodybuilder. I'm not saying organic, no gmo's, no gluten is the way to go I'm just saying eat like a bodybuilder look like a bodybuilder and you can perform like a strength athlete. This approach does require some self control which isn't easy for powerlifters   as we always take things to the extreme but I feel that this is not only the healthier route but it will also be the route that will give you the best strength result.

With the cyclic carb approach you go on a week to week basis if weight is moving up don't change a thing if it starts to stale add 10% to your carbs, start around the workout first then partition them downwards. Keep this up until it stales again then up your fats by 10%, note that any subject lines with a zero should stay that way. The constant rotation of the days should be enough to never overstimulate your insulin receptors to the point where you become insulin resistant. This means that if you are constantly spiking your insulin daily your receptor cells become less likely to store carbs into muscle glycogen and start storing them into fat cells because food has to go somewhere no matter what and if you're constantly over doing things they will normally go straight to fat cells.

This approach albeit healthy does require a mini diet of sorts as well. You can run the above cyclic approach for anywhere from 16-20 weeks and a 4 week mini diet, rinse and repeat. The reason for mini diets in both cases is to minimize fat gain and to desensitize your body to carbs again, your body can only take in so many carbs for an extended time before you become insulin resistant so instead of carbs shuttling all your nutrients to glycogen stores and muscle tissue it will start to store it as fat so your fat cells will continue to grow and you'll stop adding muscle and just get all soft and fluffy.

Remember muscle contracts and moves weight not fat, fat just changes your leverages and can make you stronger in that instance but it may also affect your lifts as well. Have you ever seen a super fat guy squat and deadlift its just ugly let alone you should   always be able to bend over and tie your own shoe without passing out. Although we go to great extremes to be the best at our sport, some things shouldn't be compromised, but that's debatable.

Now that we got bulking out of the way and laid a lot of the general principles down throughout this book, the cutting section won't be that long, but if you decide to embark on it, I promise you it will be tedious and tough. Most people reading this will either be looking for simple guidance on how to lose weight, eat better,   or   maximize   performance.   If performance is what you're after than a lot of times   it   comes   down   to   maximizing performance in a certain weight class and since fat doesn't move weight its best to be the leanest and most muscular guy or girl in your desired weight class.

Now before we get into the in and outs of cutting let me first say that as a beginner meaning 1-4 years of experience lifting you should just focus on getting as big and as strong as you can be with proper nutrition and training. After you have put in some time than and only than I would think about cutting down some body fat and getting to a more competitive weight class.

As a strength athlete I only recommend being in a calorie deficit for maximum 12 weeks weeks, for general population as long as it takes to reach your goals is fine. Once you have your maintenance balance of calories established, which remember may take 2-3 weeks, you can start the leaning out process. The worst thing you can do is start out with extremely low calories and extremely high cardio this will give you an initial weight loss but will mess things up for the rest of the cut. Because you will hit a plateau and once you do you have two options either lower calories even more or raise cardio even higher. So my basic philosophy in leaning out is to get as much out of doing as little as possible. Meaning if we set a diet and weight is coming off than there is absolutely no need to add any cardio or make any adjustments until we plateau again.

Let the food do the work and keeping calories as high as possible will help keep your metabolism burning and allowing for constant steady progress. I also don't add in any cardio until the first plateau, once you hit the first of many I keep calories the same and add in more work either another day of training or starting up some cardio. What we do on a day to day basis from the stand point of energy expenditure is what keeps our metabolism burning so doing more and keeping food high is ideal.

Where to begin when we start dumping calories to help in our weight loss journey is easy we first eliminate 5% of our daily amounts of fat. Fat being 9 calories per gram is an easy fix to get the balance tipping in the negative again so progress can continue.

After that adjustment is made we ride it out until another plateau is hit than we take out 5% of total daily carbohydrates except for the ones pre, during, and post workout. Two things to consider when dieting is one protein never gets change and the last bit of carbohydrates taken out of the diet will be in this order intra workout carbs is the absolute last, post workout carbs next, and pre workout carbs first but make sure all other carbs besides those are eliminated first. Once you make a reduction in the two macronutrients the next thing to adjust is work and you just simply add more, either adding in another day of cardio or 5 minutes extra per day of cardio. It's that simple in the 3 months of dieting you just make these minor adjustments when stuck to see major gains by the end. Once you are done with the diet I highly recommend adding in 5% of your calories weekly split up how you like because by now you have a good understanding of what macros fit you best and how your body responds and at the end of 6-8 weeks of this you decide whether to cut again or start a bulk.

CHAPTER 8: RECOVER AND GROW

The ability to recover fast from workouts is key to continuing to make gains and grow week to week. Recovery is not only how well you recover day to day, but also you ability to withstand more and more on a week to week basis as you up the intensity, frequency, and volume. Some key factors to aid in recovery are:

- Sleep
- Proper Programming
- Nutrition
- Restoration Protocol
- Ergogenic Aids/Supplements
- Managing Stress

Sleep is extremely important in that it

helps your body regulate back to normal functions, it helps reset and bring down stress levels aka cortisol, helps with GH release, and adapt to the training stimulus. 8-10 hours is ideal for an athlete along with 15-20 min power naps throughout the day. You want to keep the naps short in duration as a longer nap will stimulate sleep inertia, which is a period after the nap that impairs performance and alertness.

Researcher Cheri Mah of the Stanford Sleep Disorders Clinic and Research Laboratory has studied the effects of sleep and athletic performance. Mah noted that sleep is a "significant factor in achieving peak athletic performance." Mah continued that many athletes accumulate a large sleep debt by not obtaining their required nightly sleep, which can have a negative effects on cognitive functioning, mood, and reaction time. Not surprisingly though, Mah's suggested that the "negative effects can be minimized or eliminated by prioritizing sleep in general and, more specifically, obtaining extra sleep aka naps to reduce one's sleep debt." This sleep debt can't be made up with one good night of sleep it takes weeks to turn it back around.

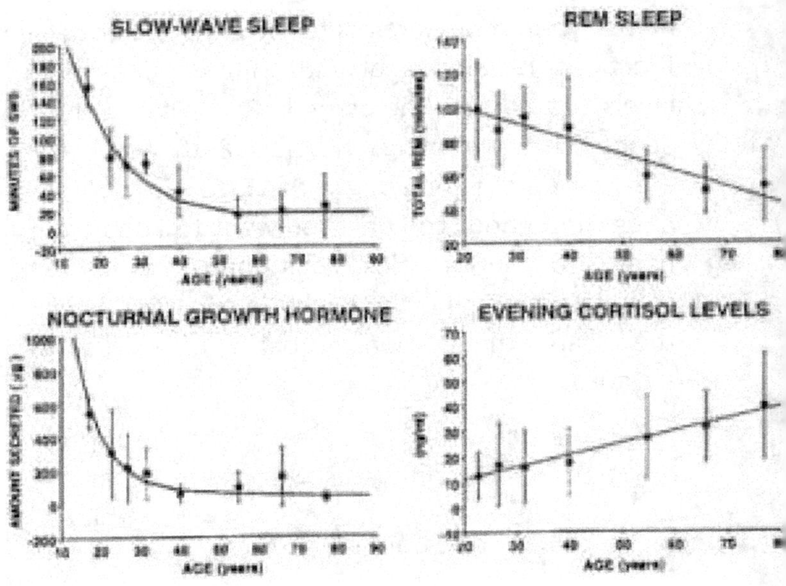

A few simple things to improve sleep are blackout curtains which you can get at Walmart, removing all electronics from your room, having a bedtime routine routine, staying away from TV or loud action packed things that will elevate your heart rate, read a book that doesn't get your mind racing, and a little meditation which is invaluable in and of itself.

Proper programming is huge in your ability to recover from a day to day perspective. To much volume and intensity and you'll lead to overtraining, injury, and to much fatigue which will all lead to a decrease in performance. The ability to understand programming and waving intensities and volume to allow for proper recover in bet training days is huge to progressing forward. Not going to failure everyday is very important as well, failure training can be ok if implemented right but when it comes to your main lifts failure should never be an option. Planning out your days and weeks based on wave loading principals is a great way to allow for proper recover. An example of this would be to have a hypertrophy day where nothing is taking above a RPE of 7, followed up with a heavy day where the RPE is an 8 but with no missed reps so a technical RPE 8 not a grinder, follow that up with some more dynamic movements learning to move weight fast and controlled with a RPE 6. Waving your days or sessions like this will help auto regulate in a way your intensity and volume to allow for proper recovery.

Nutrition is a component in recovery and sports for that matter that is often overlooked. Some will go with the war on carbs, or eat whatever I can, or intermittent fasting, etc.. The key with nutrition is knowing why and what it is used for and the benefits of everything you put into your body. Workouts will deplete your body and the best way to refill it is by eating carbohydrates around your workout. Workouts also breakdown muscle tissue and if not fueled with enough protein they won't recover properly. Workouts also build up cortisol and can cause havoc on your joints and hormones, so eating your fats throughout the day will help bring everything back to a normal status. Gaining to much fat will also slow down recover as it is not optimal for your body to be to fat or to lean. The biggest key to improvement in recovery and performance from a nutrition stand point is to

- Almost never be in an extended calorie deficit
- Don't skip any of the macros
- Eat the right amount of protein for your bodyweight
- Time your carbohydrates around your workouts

Having a recovery/restoration protocol in place will do wonders for your body, mind, and spirit. When all 3 of those are in perfect harmony great things can happen on the platform or in the gym. This is also often overlooked in its importance to an athlete. It starts with a proper warm up before the workout, nothing crazy just something to get the blood flowing. An example would be:

5 minutes on bike
5 minutes pulling a sled
10 minutes of a dynamic warm up Possible Effects

of an Active Warm Up

- Increased resistance of muscle and joints
- Increased release of oxygen from hemoglobin and myoglobin
- Increased rate of metabolic reactions
- Increased nerve conduction rate
- Increased blood flow to muscles
- Increased speed and force of muscle contractions
- Increased baselineoxygcen consumption

*Bishop, D. Warm up II: performance changes following active warm up and how to structure the warm up. *Sports Med 33:483-498, 2003*

Make sure the dynamic warm up is in conjunction with the exercises that will be lifted that day and try to avoid a lot of foam rolling and static stretching at this time. As this has been shown to decrease performance.

A cool down is just as important as a warm up. It will allow your body to get blood flowing for muscle repair, discard waste, and to replenish energy in a less intensive manner that will help start the recovery process at a rapid pace. A cool down is a great time to also work on flexibility with some light static stretching and a light massage with either a foam roller or barbell.

After the workout is done and leading into the next workout things such as massage, hot/cold therapy, sauna and muscle stimulation can all be used to help with the day in and day out recovery process. All these modalities are great for restoration, stress relief, reduction of anxiety, tension, stress, and depression; improves mood, and an increase in well being.*My good friend Brandon Allen always tells me recover harder than you train and he was right as usual.

*Weinber, R. A. Jackson, and K. Kolodny, The relationship of massage and exercise to mood enhancement. *Sports Psychol 2:202-211 1988*

Ergogenic aids and supplements can also play a big role in recovery. The use of steroids has a huge role in the recovery process, but also can have some side affects   so always consult with a Dr. before taking anything of that nature. Supplements can also aid in recovery, whether it be in the form of a sleep aid or the form of a peri workout   drink. Sleep aids can help you get deeper and fuller sleep which as stated above is an awesome way to promote recovery. Periworkout drinks can also help in several ways but the 2 most important is the blunting of muscle breakdown during the workout and   the increase in protein synthesis post workout. Drinking a fast digesting carb and whey protein mixed with some bcaa's will do the trick in helping you power through a workout with better energy and it will help diminish the catabolic effect of a hard workout on the muscles.

A ratio of 4:1 carbohydrates to protein is an ideal ratio for the periworkout shake. So if you consume 25g of protein you'll consume 100g of carbohydrates. Not only will this rink help with muscle repair, insulin spike, gh release, it will increase your work capacity during the training session.*

*Ivy, J. and R. Portman, The future of sports nutrition: Nutrient timing. North Bergen, NJ: Basic Health; 2004

Stress management is a component of recovery that nobody talks about. Life will always be there it will have ups and downs and being able to manage that will help performance improve tremendously. Ways of coping with stress will be different for everyone, but some recommended ways to deal with it is from meditation, reading, breathing, massage, exercise and writing.

Stress is simply the body's response to changes that create taxing demands. There are

2 types of stress Eustress which is positive and distress which is negative. Distress is always going to be around learning to cope with it will allow you to keep moving forward in training and in life. Stress prevention is basically about cultivating a balanced perspective towards one's life and place within the world. Generally speaking, the following steps will allow people to reduce stress:

- becoming aware of what true needs are and are not
- understanding how to meet true needs (rejecting mere wishes masquerading as true needs)
- becoming able to resist being exploited or manipulated by other people

Efforts to clarify values, ambitions and social boundaries; to become aware of physical limitations and meet basic needs; to recognize and fend off interpersonal exploitation and invasion; and to cultivate a positive, optimistic and emotionally resilient attitude towards life are all important aspects of developing this perspective.*

*Harry Mills, Ph.D., Natalie Reiss, Ph.D. and Mark Dombeck, Ph.D. sevencounties.org

Taking your recovery to the next step will help take your performance to the next level.

CHAPTER 9: THE GROCERY LIST

What good is all this information if you don't know what to eat. I've put together a list of recommended foods. Now with that being said I am sure i missed some foods so   if you eat something not on the list just make sure it adheres to the logic and macros presented above.

Lean Protein (especially on high carb days)
Boneless Skinless Chicken Breast Tilapia
Cod Halibut
Extra Lean Ground Turkey Egg Whites

Fattier Protein
Chicken Thighs
Lean Ground Beef 90/10 or better Filet Mignon

Flank Steak
Top Round Steak Salmon
Tuna
Lean Turkey Breast

Carbohydrates Complex
Brown Rice
Brown Rice Pasta
Oatmeal
Sweet Potatoes
Ezekial Bread
Couscous
Quinoa
Cream of Wheat
Squash
Zucchini

Carbohydrates Simple

White Jasmine Rice
White Potato
Rice Cakes Cream of Rice Fruit (minimal) HBCD
Karbolyn

Carbohydrates Refeed Day

Low Fat Pancakes /w Syrup
Low Fat Sugary Cereal /w Skim Milk
Fat Free Frozen Yogurt
Snack Wells
Low Fat Low Fat Pop Tarts
Low Fat Baked Goods
Low Fat Graham Crackers

Fats
Coconut Oil
Extra Virgin
Olive Oil
Natural Nut Butters
Sharp or Aged Cheese
Grass Fed Butter
Avocado
Mixed Nuts
Fish Oil
Borage Oil
MCT Oil

Vegetables
Asparagus
Broccoli
Cauliflower
Spinach
Romaine Lettuce
Green Beans
Brussel Sprouts